BATTLING COVID-19

Leaders
TAKE CHARGE

Guiding the Nation through COVID-19

RACHAEL L. THOMAS

Checkerboard
Library

An Imprint of Abdo Publishing
abdobooks.com

abdobooks.com

Published by Abdo Publishing, a division of ABDO, PO Box 398166, Minneapolis, Minnesota 55439. Copyright © 2021 by Abdo Consulting Group, Inc. International copyrights reserved in all countries. No part of this book may be reproduced in any form without written permission from the publisher. Checkerboard Library™ is a trademark and logo of Abdo Publishing.

Printed in the United States of America, North Mankato, Minnesota
102020
012021

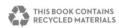
THIS BOOK CONTAINS
RECYCLED MATERIALS

Design: Sarah DeYoung, Mighty Media, Inc.
Production: Mighty Media, Inc.
Editor: Jessica Rusick
Cover Photograph: Bloomberg/Getty Images
Interior Photographs: AP Images, p. 9; Chia-Chi Charlie Chang/NIH/Flickr, p. 29; Keith Allison/Wikimedia Commons, p. 7; Nestor Galina/Flickr, pp. 6 (bottom), 11; Shutterstock Images, pp. 5, 6, 16, 17, 21, 25; Ted S. Warren/AP Images, p. 19; The White House/Flickr, pp. 13, 26; Wilson Ring/AP Images, p. 23
Design Elements: Shutterstock Images

Library of Congress Control Number: 2020940253

Publisher's Cataloging-in-Publication Data
Names: Thomas, Rachael L., author.
Title: Leaders take charge: guiding the nation through COVID-19 / by Rachael L. Thomas
Other title: guiding the nation through COVID-19
Description: Minneapolis, Minnesota : Abdo Publishing, 2021 | Series: Battling COVID-19 | Includes online resources and index
Identifiers: ISBN 9781532194306 (lib. bdg.) | ISBN 9781098213664 (ebook)
Subjects: LCSH: COVID-19 (Disease)--Juvenile literature. | Presidents--Juvenile literature. | Center for Disease Control--Juvenile literature. | Governors--Juvenile literature. | Communicable diseases—Prevention—Juvenile literature.
Classification: DDC 920.00904--dc23

Contents

An Invisible Threat

In December 2019, people across the world turned their attention to the city of Wuhan, China. Citizens there were becoming **infected** with a dangerous new coronavirus. This virus caused a disease called COVID-19. Many people were falling ill.

New COVID-19 cases soon began appearing outside of China. In late January, the United States reported its first case. At the time, little was known about the virus that caused COVID-19. Scientists were still learning how it made people sick.

On March 11, 2020, the **World Health Organization (WHO)** declared COVID-19 a **pandemic**. Nobody was sure how far COVID-19 might spread. And, nobody knew how to cure it. In the meantime, leaders in the United States and around the world had to make difficult decisions. And to save lives, they had to act fast.

WHAT IS A CORONAVIRUS?

Coronaviruses are a large group of viruses that cause **respiratory** illnesses. Most coronaviruses exist only in animals. However, several have spread from animals to humans. The coronavirus discovered in Wuhan is called severe acute respiratory syndrome coronavirus 2 (SARS-CoV-2). It causes a disease called coronavirus disease 2019, or COVID-19. COVID-19 spreads when saliva droplets pass from person to person. This can happen when someone coughs, sneezes, sings, breathes, or talks. Most people with COVID-19 do not suffer serious **symptoms**. But some people develop life-threatening problems. Because of this, the virus is viewed as a threat to world health.

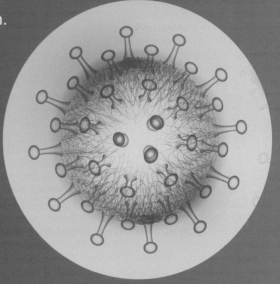

TIMELINE

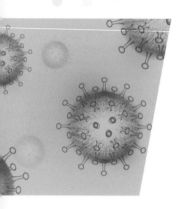

DECEMBER 16, 2019

One of the earliest known COVID-19 patients is hospitalized in China.

JANUARY 21, 2020

The first US case of COVID-19 is reported.

MARCH 5, 2020

Technology company Microsoft encourages employees to work from home.

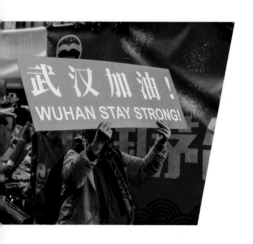

武汉加油!
WUHAN STAY STRONG!

JANUARY 23, 2020

The city of Wuhan, China, is ordered into lockdown.

JANUARY 29, 2020

President Trump announces the White House Coronavirus Task Force.

MARCH 27, 2020

President Trump signs the Coronavirus Aid, Relief, and Economic Security (CARES) Act into law.

MARCH 11, 2020

The World Health Organization (WHO) declares COVID-19 a pandemic.

APRIL 16, 2020

The US government releases guidelines advising states on how to reopen.

MARCH 11, 2020

National Basketball League Commissioner Adam Silver postpones the 2020 basketball season.

OCTOBER 2, 2020

President Trump announces that he has COVID-19.

EARLY JUNE 2020

Most US states have started reopening.

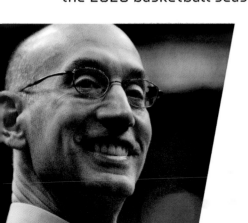

7

A Secretive Start

One of China's earliest known COVID-19 patients was hospitalized on December 16, 2019. Chinese officials reported the **outbreak** to the **WHO** on December 31. But the government was slow to release other information to world health officials. So in those first weeks, Chinese authorities mostly faced the COVID-19 threat alone.

At first, Chinese authorities tried to suppress news of the disease. In the meantime, Chinese scientists studied the virus. They took samples of the virus from **infected** patients. This helped the scientists learn more about it.

On January 11, 2020, China announced that its scientists had mapped the virus's **genome**. Scientists around the world used the genome to produce COVID-19 tests. These tests determine if someone has COVID-19.

By the time of the announcement, more than three weeks had passed since China's first COVID-19 hospitalization. But the government had not yet warned the public about the dangers of COVID-19. So, the disease continued to spread.

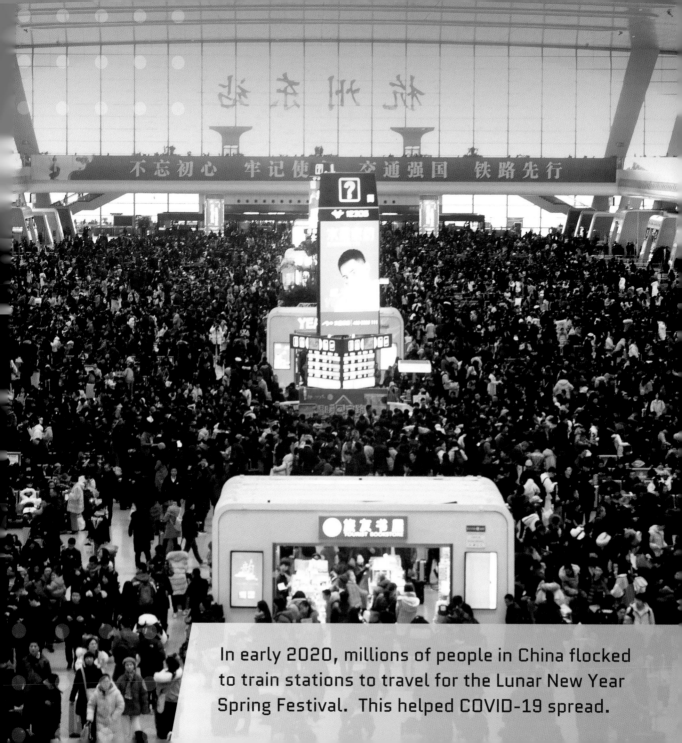

In early 2020, millions of people in China flocked to train stations to travel for the Lunar New Year Spring Festival. This helped COVID-19 spread.

STEM CONNECTION

Handshakes are an important custom in many Western cultures. But a person's palm can carry many germs. These germs can be transferred to another person during a handshake. So, many leaders stopped shaking hands during the **pandemic**. They bowed instead.

By late January, COVID-19 cases began to appear in nearby countries. Chinese authorities were forced to act. The city of Wuhan went into **lockdown** on January 23. Many businesses closed. These included schools and restaurants.

The lockdown also banned travel to and from Wuhan. Residents were ordered to leave home only for food and medicine. And, authorities **quarantined** people **infected** with COVID-19. On January 24, China's Prime Minister Xi Jinping expanded the lockdown. Other parts of China were now affected. Tens of millions of people were confined to their homes.

Experts later agreed that China's lockdown slowed the spread of COVID-19. But critics said China's government should have warned the public about the disease sooner. This could have prevented thousands of infections.

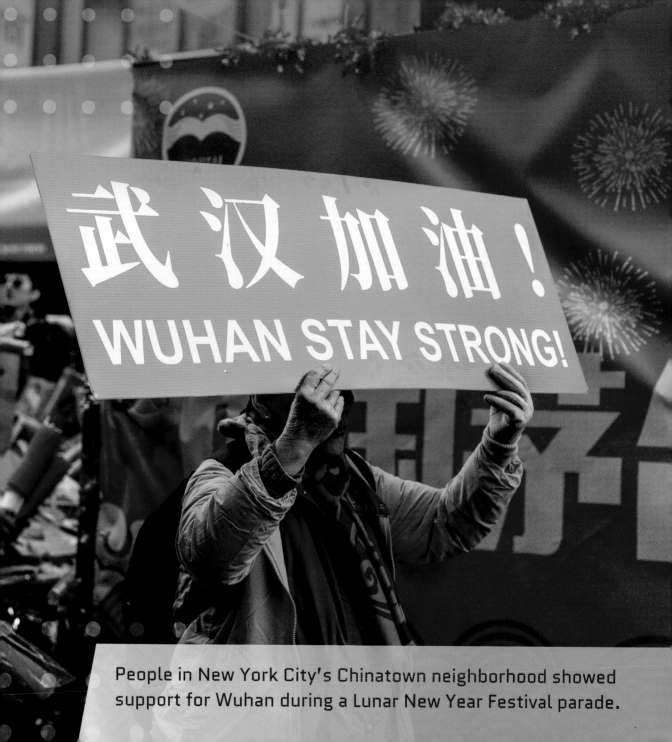

武汉加油！
WUHAN STAY STRONG!

People in New York City's Chinatown neighborhood showed
support for Wuhan during a Lunar New Year Festival parade.

Arrival in the US

Despite Wuhan's **lockdown**, COVID-19 spread to countries overseas. The US reported its first case of COVID-19 on January 21, 2020. On January 29, President Donald Trump announced the White House Coronavirus Task Force. The task force would lead the government's response to the virus.

The task force included leaders from several government departments and health agencies. One leader was Dr. Anthony Fauci. Fauci was the Director of the National Institute of Allergy and **Infectious** Diseases. He had advised several US presidents on global health issues.

On January 31, the task force declared COVID-19 a national public health emergency. That same day, the US government banned all travel from Wuhan to the United States.

By the end of January, fewer than ten Americans had been **diagnosed** with COVID-19. Much was still unknown about the disease. Despite this, American leaders felt sure that COVID-19 was under control. President Trump also did not want the public to panic over the disease. So, he told the nation not to worry.

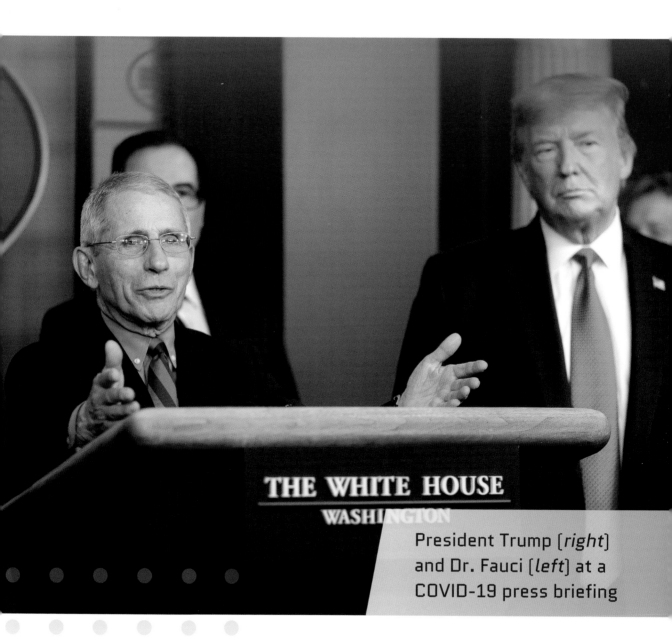

President Trump [*right*] and Dr. Fauci [*left*] at a COVID-19 press briefing

The Lost Month

In February, the number of COVID-19 cases rose across the world. By the end of the month, China had almost 80,000 cases. Italy had more than 1,000.

In the United States, reported COVID-19 cases rose to 25 during February. These reported numbers were low. So, federal and state leaders took little action against the disease.

However, the reported numbers were **inaccurate**. This was due to issues with testing. One issue was that a new test developed by the **Centers for Disease Control and Prevention (CDC)** did not work correctly. It took weeks to fix the test and then the US government was slow to expand testing.

Another issue was that few people had access to tests. That meant many cases of COVID-19 were not officially counted. So, experts believe the United States had many more cases than were being reported.

Critics of the US **pandemic** response would later call February 2020 a "lost month." They said the US government should have expanded COVID-19 testing in February to help contain COVID-19.

WHY PRACTICE SOCIAL DISTANCING?

Social Distancing

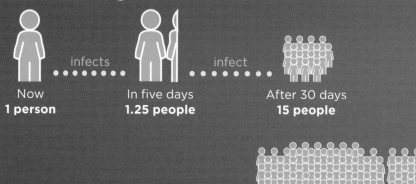

Now	In five days	After 30 days
1 person	**1.25 people**	**15 people**

No Social Distancing

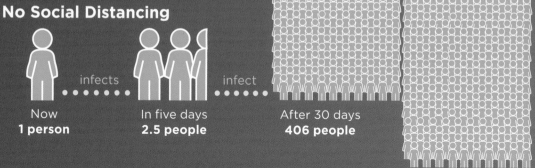

Now	In five days	After 30 days
1 person	**2.5 people**	**406 people**

On March 15, the **CDC** recommended that people practice social distancing. This would limit the spread of COVID-19. Social distancing meant staying at least six feet (2 m) away from others. It also meant avoiding large gatherings. Social distancing limited people's interactions with one another. This resulted in fewer people becoming **infected** with COVID-19 over time.

Global Impact

DENMARK

On March 13, Denmark's president, Mette Frederiksen, closed the country's borders. Days later, she closed the country's schools. She also banned gatherings of more than ten people. Frederiksen's early actions limited COVID-19's spread. So, Denmark had fewer COVID-19 cases than many other European countries.

IRELAND

Ireland's prime minister, Dr. Leo Varadkar, imposed a national **lockdown** in late March. The lockdown banned most **nonessential** travel within the country. Varadkar was a former doctor. So, he assisted medical workers in Ireland's hospitals during the **crisis**.

TAIWAN

Taiwan's first COVID-19 case was reported on January 21. President Tsai Ing-wen soon began mapping the travel of **infected** individuals. This helped the government track how and where COVID-19 was spreading. Ing-wen's leadership kept the number of cases in Taiwan low.

NEW ZEALAND

On March 23, New Zealand's prime minister, Jacinda Ardern, ordered a **lockdown**. At the time, New Zealand had only 102 COVID-19 cases. The lockdown closed all but **essential** businesses. Ardern's actions helped keep the country's case numbers low.

States Respond

In early March, Americans were still living as normal. However, some state officials were beginning to worry about COVID-19. Ohio, Washington, and California had already had COVID-19 **outbreaks**. So, state leaders introduced protective measures to stop the disease's spread.

On March 12, Ohio governor Mike DeWine ordered schools in the state to close. On March 15, Washington governor Jay Inslee signed an emergency declaration. It closed restaurants and other businesses in the state. On March 16, California governor Gavin Newsom ordered **nonessential** businesses in the state to close. Three days later, he ordered California residents to stay home.

FIGHTING DISCRIMINATION

Asians and people of Asian descent faced **discrimination** during the **pandemic**. This is because COVID-19 emerged in Asia. Governments sometimes fueled this behavior. Several leaders made anti-Asian comments during the pandemic. Human rights groups encouraged world leaders to stop anti-Asian abuse.

Most states were not yet acting against COVID-19. Many leaders still felt the disease was not a threat. For example, the mayor of New York City encouraged people to gather normally. This was despite growing public concern over the virus.

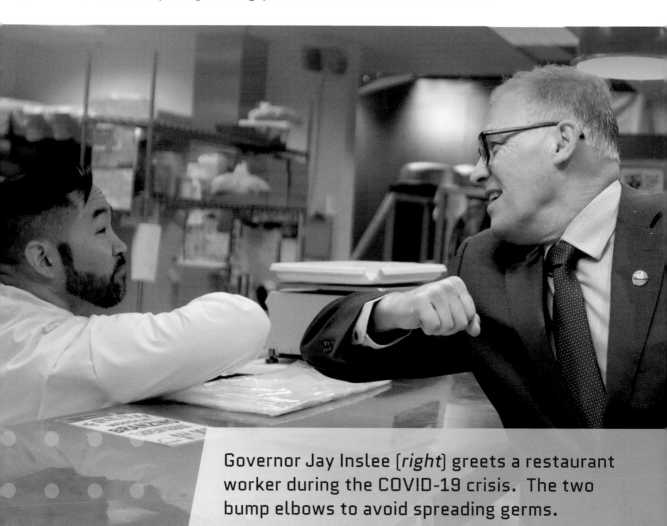

Governor Jay Inslee (*right*) greets a restaurant worker during the COVID-19 crisis. The two bump elbows to avoid spreading germs.

However, New York soon became a global center of the COVID-19 **pandemic**. By mid-March, the state was reporting thousands of new COVID-19 **infections** each day. New York had the worst COVID-19 **outbreak** in the United States.

On March 20, New York governor Andrew Cuomo issued a statewide stay-at-home order. Under this order, people were asked to only leave their homes for necessary travel. This included buying food and medicine. In addition, only **essential** businesses could remain open. These included grocery stores and hospitals. Many other businesses had to close.

Cuomo earned international praise for his leadership during the **crisis**. In March, he began holding daily press briefings. Cuomo used the press briefings to give updates about the pandemic. He also talked about the struggles everyday New Yorkers faced. Some had lost loved ones to COVID-19. Many others felt **stressed** and lonely from staying at home. Cuomo's honesty earned him the trust of New Yorkers and many other Americans.

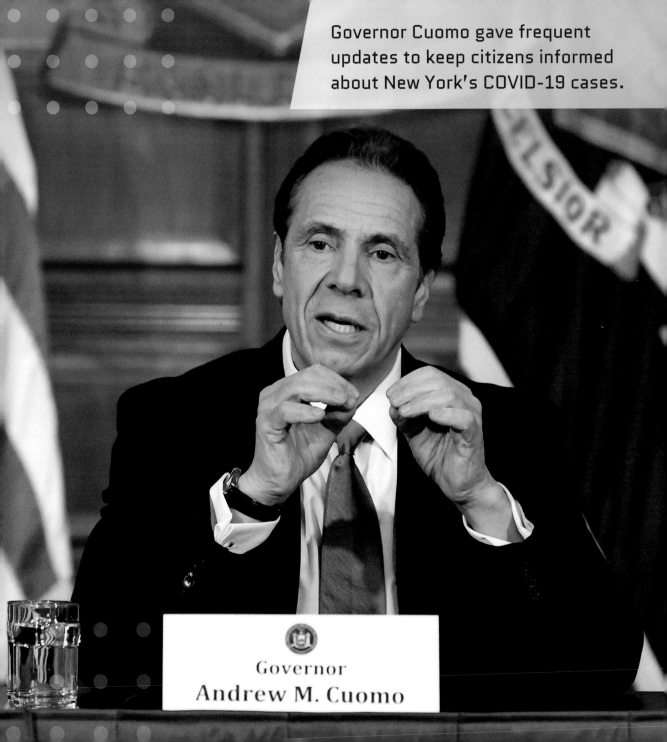

Governor Cuomo gave frequent updates to keep citizens informed about New York's COVID-19 cases.

Governor
Andrew M. Cuomo

Leading by Example

Government leaders played a key role during the COVID-19 **crisis.** But other public figures helped deliver important information. Singers such as Taylor Swift and Lady Gaga used social media to encourage social distancing. They posted pictures of themselves working from home and wearing face masks.

Business leaders carried influence too. On March 5, technology company Microsoft encouraged its employees to work from home. Other businesses soon followed Microsoft's lead.

Sports organizations also made important decisions. One organization to act early was the National Basketball Association (NBA). On March 11, NBA Commissioner Adam Silver **postponed** the NBA's season. This prevented people from spreading COVID-19

STEM CONNECTION

In early April, the **CDC** recommended that people wear face masks in public. These helped reduce the spread of COVID-19. The masks help contain droplets we exhale when we talk, cough, or sneeze. These droplets carry germs, including the ones that cause COVID-19.

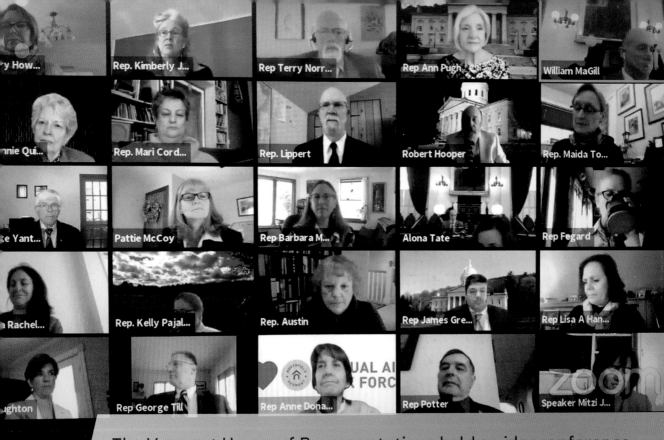

The Vermont House of Representatives held a videoconference in April. These types of meetings allowed local government leaders to pass bills during the crisis.

at crowded games. Other sports leagues soon **postponed** their seasons as well. Some sports eventually returned over the summer. However, teams often played in empty stadiums. This helped keep fans and players safe.

The Response Continues

By April 1, the United States had more than 200,000 COVID-19 cases. State and local leaders continued responding to the **crisis**. By April 7, most state governors had issued stay-at-home orders.

Stay-at-home orders helped keep COVID-19 from spreading. However, as businesses closed, millions of people lost their jobs. And, businesses that remained open were not making as much money. Many struggled to pay their employees.

So, the US federal government passed legislation to provide relief to Americans. On March 27, President Trump signed the Coronavirus Aid, Relief, and Economic Security (CARES) Act into law. The CARES Act dedicated $2.2 trillion to supporting the US economy. This included $350 billion to help small businesses pay their employees.

The act also included $140 billion for hospitals and healthcare workers. The money gave healthcare workers protective

COVID-19 INFECTIONS BY STATE
(DECEMBER 2020)

| 1,001-10,000 CASES | 10,001-100,000 CASES | 100,001-500,000 CASES | MORE THAN 500,000 CASES |

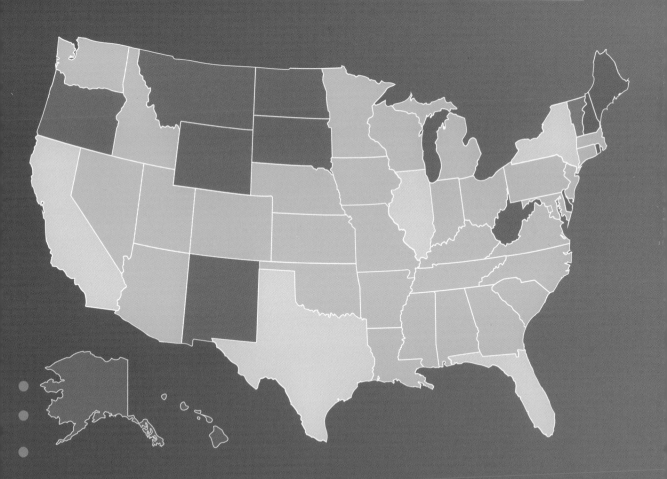

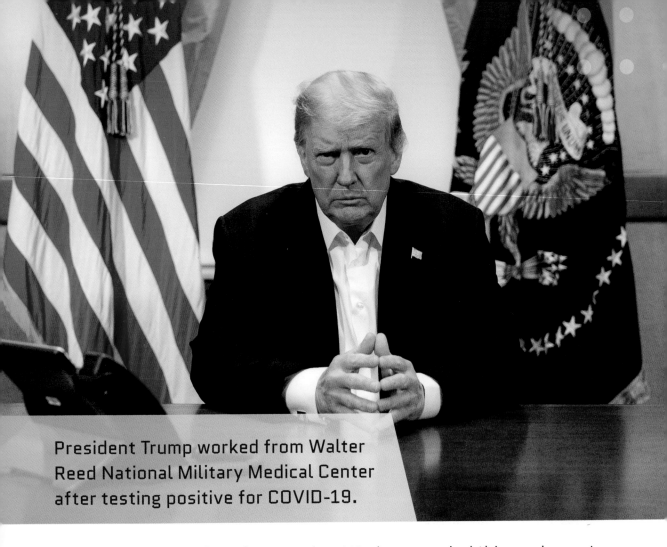

President Trump worked from Walter Reed National Military Medical Center after testing positive for COVID-19.

equipment, such as face masks. Workers needed this equipment to safely treat COVID-19 patients.

People worried about the economic effects of the **pandemic**. Some were eager for stay-at-home orders to end and state economies to reopen. Others were worried that cases would increase if states reopened too quickly. On April 16, the US government released reopening guidelines. These guidelines offered suggestions for how states could slowly and safely reopen.

By early June, most states had started reopening. Many businesses had safety measures in place such as limiting the number of people in a building at one time. And, many state leaders still encouraged social distancing in public.

Later that month, case numbers began to increase. States with the highest increases included California, Texas, and Florida. Governors in these states chose to pause or reverse reopening.

Meanwhile, the 2020 presidential election was approaching. The **pandemic** was a key issue. President Trump and his opponent, Joe Biden, had different views on the **crisis**. Trump said the pandemic would soon be over. Biden said Trump had not taken the pandemic seriously.

On October 2, President Trump announced that he had COVID-19. The same day, he went to Walter Reed National Military Medical Center for treatment. Trump left the medical center on October 5. He continued to lead the nation as he recovered.

Facing Future Challenges

The COVID-19 **pandemic** was a global **crisis.** By October 2020, tens of millions of people worldwide had been **infected** by the virus. More than 1 million had died. In the United States alone, more than 7 million people had been infected. More than 200,000 had died.

Leaders across the world had to make difficult decisions during the crisis. These decisions made some people angry. In the United States, some felt the federal government had not done enough to protect Americans from COVID-19. Other people protested that stay-at-home orders set by local leaders were too **restrictive**. But, as the pandemic wore on, American leaders continued to make the decisions they felt were best.

Current leaders have learned a lot from the COVID-19 pandemic. Leaders of tomorrow will also apply knowledge gained during the crisis. Because of this, the world will be better prepared for unexpected challenges in the future.

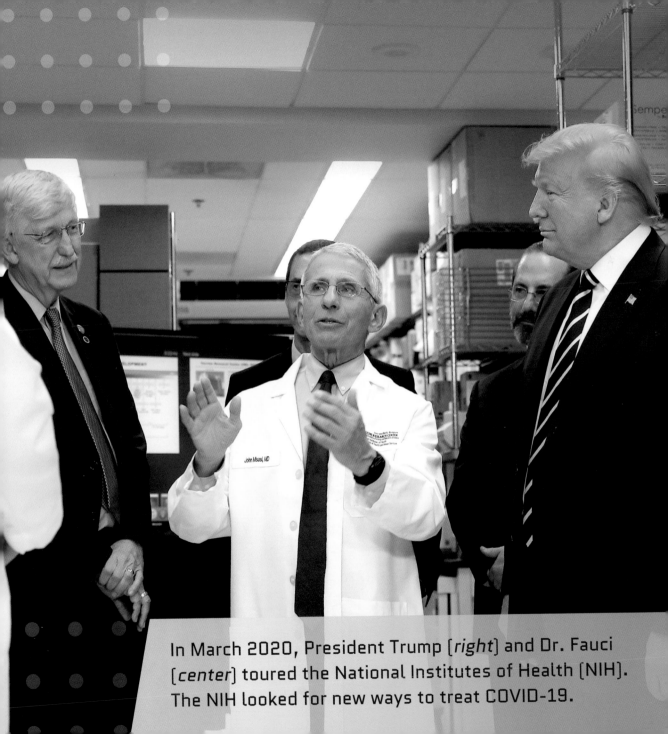

In March 2020, President Trump [*right*] and Dr. Fauci [*center*] toured the National Institutes of Health [NIH]. The NIH looked for new ways to treat COVID-19.

Glossary

Centers for Disease Control and Prevention (CDC)—the main national health organization in the United States. The CDC works to control the spread of disease and maintain and improve public health in the United States and other countries.

crisis—a difficult or dangerous situation that needs serious attention.

diagnose—to recognize something, such as a disease, by signs, symptoms, or tests.

discrimination (dihs-krih-muh-NAY-shuhn)—unfair treatment, often based on race, religion, or gender.

essential—very important or necessary. Something that is not essential is nonessential.

genome—the genetic material of an organism.

inaccurate—not precise or correct.

infection—an unhealthy condition caused by something harmful, such as a virus. If something has an infection, it is infected. Something that causes an infection is infectious.

lockdown—a temporary measure ordered by government officials in which people are required to stay at home and limit public contact.

outbreak—a sudden increase in the occurrence of an illness.

pandemic—worldwide spread of a disease that can affect most people.

postpone—to put off until a later time.

quarantine—to separate from others in order to stop a disease from spreading.

respiratory—having to do with the system of organs involved with breathing.

restrictive—limiting or controlling.

stressed—feeling a physical, chemical, or emotional factor that causes bodily or mental strain. Stress may be involved in causing some diseases.

symptom—a noticeable change in the normal working of the body. A symptom indicates or accompanies disease, sickness, or another malfunction.

World Health Organization (WHO)—an agency of the United Nations that works to maintain and improve the health of people around the world.

Online Resources

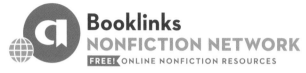

Booklinks
NONFICTION NETWORK
FREE! ONLINE NONFICTION RESOURCES

To learn more about the COVID-19 pandemic, please visit **abdobooklinks.com** or scan this QR code. These links are routinely monitored and updated to provide the most current information available.

Index